Fall Prevention:

Don't Let Your House Kick You Out!

The companion to
Fall Prevention: Stay on Your Own Two Feet!

Fall Prevention Advisors, LLC
Gail Davies, PT, GCS
Fran Scully, PT

Illustrations by Pam Gosner

ISBN 978-0-7414-3113-4

Illustrations by Pam Gosner, no illustrations are to be copied or sold. All rights reserved.

Published by:

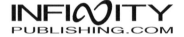
PUBLISHING.COM

Info@buybooksontheweb.com
www.buybooksontheweb.com
Toll-free (877) BUY BOOK
Local Phone (610) 941-9999
Fax (610) 941-9959

Printed in the United States of America

Published October 2012

Introduction

Are you at risk for a fall?
1 in 3 adults over 65 fall each year.

Are your parents at risk for a fall?
The risk of falling increases exponentially with age.

Is your home a fall hazard?
Two-thirds to one-half of falls occur in and around the home.

Are you in control of where you want to live?
Nine out of ten of those 65 and older would like to remain at home.

Fall Prevention: Don't Let Your House Kick You Out! is a valuable resource for people who want to age safely at home. Physical therapists teach how to identify and eliminate fall hazards by walking the reader through an inspection of their home. Simple home modifications and helpful hints are presented.

The companion volume, *Fall Prevention: Stay on Your Own Two Feet!,* teaches how to identify and eliminate fall hot spots by walking the reader through an inspection of their body and their life. A comprehensive fall prevention program needs to address all three areas; your home, your body and your life. To be effective in preventing falls we recommend both books:

Fall Prevention: Don't Let Your House Kick You Out!

Fall Prevention: Stay On Your Own Two Feet!

Statistics reported or taken from AARP, www.aarp.org and/or CDC, www.cdc.gov

Acknowledgements

We would like to express our appreciation to all those who helped with editing, proofreading and providing professional support during the development of this book. We thank Joseph Ryan M.D. for reading and providing suggestions, Barbara Hudgins for her brain storming sessions, our editing team of June Jeannette, Jane Schroll, and Joan Temple for reading our material, and Marian Burros for sending us news clippings.

We offer a special thank you to our parents, Martha Stenard and George and Lynn Bain for their ideas and support and to our husbands and children for their encouragement throughout the development of this book.

We would like to give special acknowledgement to Pam Gosner for her tireless collaboration: in addition to being our illustrator she offered many useful suggestions.

About The Authors and Illustrator

Gail Davies has over 20 years experience as a physical therapist and is a board certified geriatric specialist. Her experience is in long term care, private practice and home care.

Fran Scully is a physical therapist. She has worked primarily in rehabilitation, geriatrics and long term care. Both authors reside in New Jersey.

The authors were motivated to write this book after treating patients with fall related injuries. They also provide education to caregivers and community groups on home modifications and strategies to prevent falls.

Their website is www.fallpreventionadvisors.com

Pam Gosner is a professional artist and former children's librarian with many years of experience creating artwork for library programs, as well as illustrating her own books on historic architecture of the West Indies.

Fall Prevention:
Don't Let Your House Kick You Out!

Table of Contents

Let's Begin!

Don't Let Your House Kick You Out!

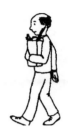

Entrance

Welcome

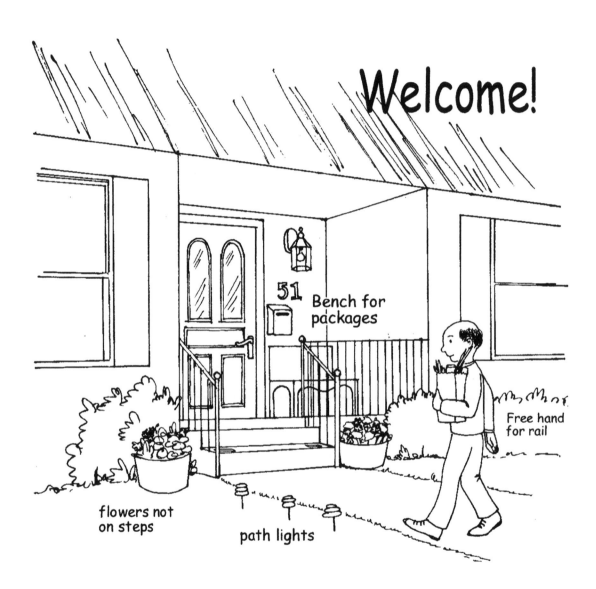

ENTRANCE

Do you have???
- level walkways
- a clear clutter free path
- a lighted path
- secure steps
- steps with highlighted edges
- clear steps
- secure hand railings
- hand railings that extend beyond the top and bottom step
- adequate lighting
- a light fixture with accessible bulbs
- an accessible mailbox
- an area to place packages
- an easily managed screen/storm door
- door knobs that can be easily opened
- locks that can be easily managed

Hot Spot
Entrance

Hot spots are:
- uneven walkways
- paths cluttered with wet leaves and grass
- flower pots on steps/walkway
- poor lighting
- steps
- no railings
- wobbly railings
- poor access to curbside mailbox
- no place to put packages
- a cumbersome screen/storm door
- difficult doorknobs
- difficult locks

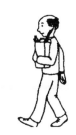

**Solution
Entrance**

1. Repair walkways.
- check walkways for heaving
- maintain level walkways
- repair wobbly steps

2. Clear walkways.
- remove leaves, grass, snow and ice
- keep ice melt by the front and back door ready for use
- remove flower pots from steps and pathways

3. Provide a well lit path.
- install outdoor lighting
- use maximum wattage allowed
- use sensor and motion detector lights
- use light fixtures with bulbs that are easy to change

Solution
Entrance

4. Highlight edge of steps.

- most falls occur on one or two step stairs and stairs of unequal riser height
- apply a small piece of reflective tape or spray paint the edge of the step with a white or contrasting paint
- use highlighting to identify unequal riser heights
- tape is available at local hardware stores
- over time reflective tape deteriorates and needs replacing

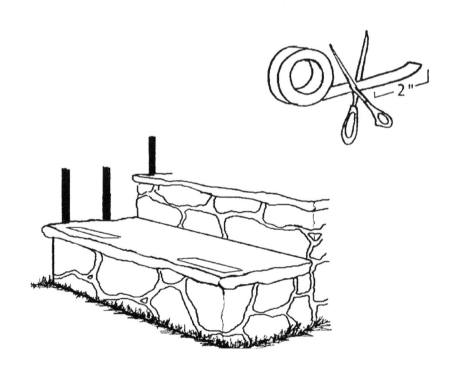

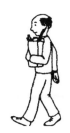

Solution
Entrance

5. Install a railing wherever there is a step.
The best hand railing is:
- rounded so it enables you to get a good grip
- at a comfortable height
- able to support your full body weight
- extends beyond the first and last step
- on both sides of the step

If you already have a railing make sure it is secure.

6. Provide safe path to mailbox.
- if needed install a railing
- roadside mailboxes should have a rear entrance for safe access to prevent stepping into the street

7. Provide easy access to front door.
- have a bench or shelf on which to place packages
- remove or replace a cumbersome screen/storm door
- replace door closure with a pneumatic closure device, located in the middle of the door; it is easier to use than having it at the bottom or top
- replace doorknobs with easy to use lever handles
- replace difficult locks with keyless pads or easy open mechanisms

Handy Gadgets

- **Key holders** enlarge the base of the key making it easier to grasp and turn

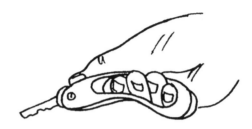

- **Lever door handles**

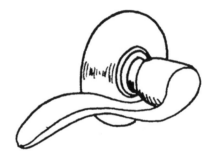

- **Motion detector and sensor lighting**
- **Keyless entry locks**
- **Ice melt** kept in closed container by front door/pathway
- **Ramp**-for every foot in elevation the ramp needs to be three feet long

Bathroom

Get a Grip

Get a Grip

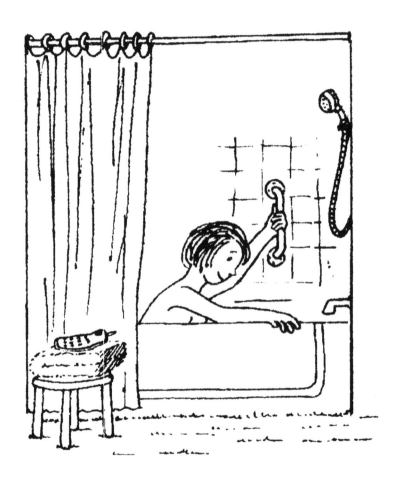

Bathroom

Are there/Is there ???

- grab bars
- cool burning night-lights
- a comfortable toilet height
- a secure toilet seat
- a slip-resistant mat or
- a slip-resistant surface on tub floor and/or shower stall floor
- a non-slip bathroom floor surface
- a hand-held shower head attached to slider bar
- a shower bench
- an accessible jacuzzi/deep tub
- an anti-scald device with hot water temperature set below 120 degrees
- an accessible phone

FYI Avoid locking the bathroom door it could delay help if you have a fall.

Hot Spot
Bathroom

Hot spots are:
- no grab bars
- loose mats
- slippery tubs/showers/floors
- loose/wobbly toilet seats
- low toilet
- poor lighting
- no phone

Philip returned from an enjoyable day of golf and now was enjoying a shower. Unfortunately, he slipped coming out of the shower and found himself on the floor. He had severe pain around his right ankle and needed his wife's support to help him to a chair. Instead of dinner, they made a trip to the local emergency room and returned hours later with an ankle cast and crutches. At least it was only a simple fracture; avoidable if all shower/bathrooms routinely included grab bars.

Solutions for Falls in the Bathroom

1. Install grab bars! Grab bars are for all ages.
- Don't be fooled. Towel bars, soap dishes, and counter tops are not a substitute for grab bars.
- Grab bars now come in decorative colors and styles. A color that contrasts with the walls is user friendly.
- For placement of grab bars check where you normally place your hands when getting in and out of the tub/shower- that place is where a grab bar needs to be. For special problems you can consult a physical or occupational therapist.
- Proper installation is necessary to ensure safety, call your handyman.

2. Get rid of slippery surfaces!
- Use slip-resistant mats inside shower/bathing area.
- Use non-slip flooring, such as wall to wall carpeting.
- Use non-slip bath mats outside tub to absorb dripping water.

3. Have a correct toilet height- raised if needed.
- Makes it easier to stand up.
- Secure any wobbly toilet seat.

4. Use non-glare lighting and cool burning night-lights.

5. Phone, a reachable phone is needed for emergencies.

Hot Spot
Deep Tubs

Jacuzzis and deep tubs can present safety problems.

Hot spots are:
- deep tubs are difficult to get in and out of
- no place for a standard grab bar
- slippery steps leading into elevated tub
- inability to get a good grip on the tub wall because of its width or shape

Joyce was perplexed after getting her new jacuzzi installed in the master bathroom. It was deep, beautifully molded and just the right shade of yellow. A wonderful air filled pillow could attach to the back with suction cups and was so comfortable to lean and relax on after an afternoon of gardening. The jacuzzi was like having a spa in her own home. Imagine her surprise when she discovered it was such a struggle to get safely out of her deep jacuzzi!

High sided claw foot round bottom tubs also present problems. If possible change to a conventional flat bottom tub, walk-in tub, or shower stall for safer entry. The expense may be well worth it.

Solutions for Getting In and Out of a Tub

1. Use a bath stool inside the tub.

Joyce now uses a small bath stool to sit on in the jacuzzi. This elevates her just enough to provide the needed leverage to enable her to get out of the tub with grace, style and safety.

2. Use a floor-to-ceiling pole.

There is a device on the market that can be used when there isn't enough wall space to accommodate a grab bar. It is a long pole that is installed from floor to ceiling and can provide a sturdy handle to hold on to when entering or exiting a deep tub or jacuzzi. (see catalogs such as AliMed in appendix)

3. Portable tub bars –Use as a guide for stepping in/out of tub. It attaches to the side of the tub, but can not be used on tubs with curved rims. Check frequently for secure fit.

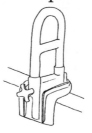

Handy Gadgets for Safer Bathrooms

- **Shower/tub bench**

There are many different models to choose from. Some are chairs with arms that go inside the tub, others have a back support and padding and then there's just a low stool. The legs are usually adjustable so you can achieve your desired sitting height. Make sure the style you choose sits flat on your tub floor. Measure tub before shopping. Today they come in delightful colors, even peacock blue.

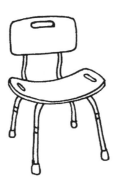

- **Hand-held Shower mounted on a sliding bar.**

A hand-held shower can be used while you sit on a shower chair. The sliding bar allows the shower head to be placed in different positions. See appendix.

- **Wingit Grab Bar Fastening System,** useful for sheet rock installation. See Sammons catalog in appendix.
- **Anti-scald device** to regulate water temperature.

- **Transfer bench**

A transfer bench is a shower bench that extends outside the tub area. There are two to four legs in the tub area (depending on the model) and two legs outside the tub. This allows you to sit on the part outside the tub area and bring your legs into the tub while sitting. If you have glass shower doors they can be easily removed.

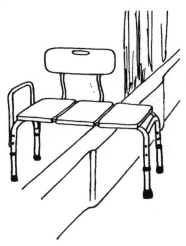

- **Walk-in Tub**

A frequently advertised bath product is a walk-in tub. It has a sealed door, molded seat and grab bar. For information see appendix.

- **Grab bars** Can be installed horizontally, vertically, or diagonally depending on your needs. Check the diameter; the most preferred are 1 to 1 1/4 inches, as they are easier to grip. A non-slip finish is desirable.

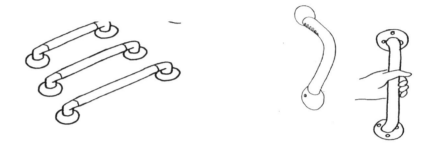

- **Elevated toilet seat**

These raise the height of the seat and enable you to sit and rise up with greater ease.

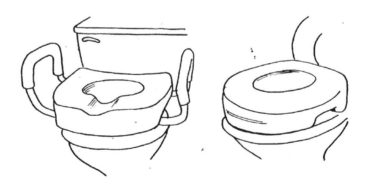

If a taller toilet fits your needs consider replacing the toilet with a "comfort height" toilet which is about two inches taller than the standard toilet.

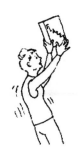

Kitchen

Know your Range of Reach

Know Your Range of Reach

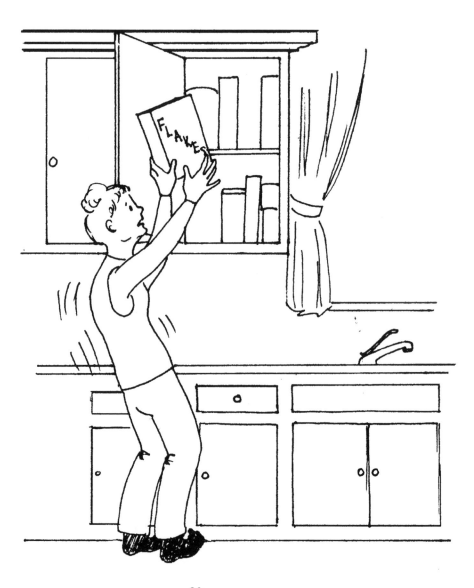

Kitchen

Are there/Is there???

- ample storage within range of reach (between waist and eye level)
- appliances at counter height
- heavy items located in low cabinets
- easily accessible major appliances
- a slip-resistant floor
- a non-slip mat in front of sink to absorb spills
- a step stool with a long handle
- an accessible fire extinguisher that you know how to use and is fully charged
- universal design

  Universal design refers to creating rooms, homes and products that can be used by everyone regardless of age, size or physical ability. If you are planning on remodeling, AARP has a free booklet on Universal Design.

Hot Spot
Reaching

To safely use a top shelf in your cupboard you need to be taller than five feet seven inches.

Hot spots are:
- items that are located too high or too low
- an overhead microwave
- cluttered cabinets
- inefficient use of counter tops
- heavy major appliance doors
- windows that are difficult to open
- spills and splashes of water and grease on the floor

Martha was reaching overhead for her cereal box when she found herself falling backward. She discovered that once a backward fall starts it is difficult to stop. She was lucky and only needed an ice bag for the bump on her head.

FYI That same backward fall can occur while trying to open a stuck double hung window or pulling on a low drawer.

Auntie Gwen was proudly carrying the duck for Christmas dinner into the dining room when we heard a thump. Auntie Gwen slipped on a splash of grease and she and the duck were on the floor. Fortunately, there were no consequences and dinner was great. She now cleans up spills as they occur.

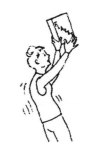

Solution for Kitchen Safety

1. Know your range of reach.
- A safe range of reach (sitting or standing) is approximately an arm's length. Use that guideline to set up your kitchen.
- Your work and storage zones should be between your waist and eye level.
- Out of range overhead storage makes the kitchen a danger zone.
- Use a reacher; see handy gadgets.
- Keep your fire extinguisher within your range of reach.

2. Use your counter tops!
- Don't be fooled by pictures in magazines, barren counter tops aren't the way to go.
- Put your coffeepot, microwave, toaster oven, mixer and blender on your counter top so they can work for you!

3. Weed out what you don't use.
- Free up your useful space, aim to stay in your range of reach.
- Store heavy items in low cabinets. If redoing the kitchen, use pull out shelves for easy access.

Solution for Kitchen Safety

4. Easily Manageable Major Appliances

- Side by side refrigerator/freezer- they allow easy access and don't have a cumbersome bottom freezer drawer.
- Don't leave pull down oven and dishwasher doors open.

One of our clients landed on her back as she did battle with her bottom freezer drawer. Steady your stance before opening a bottom freezer drawer. Have a wide base of support and place one foot ahead of the other before attempting to pull open the difficult door.

5. Step stool. Though we don't recommend climbing, we know there are times that you will.

- Don't use a chair to climb on. Invest in a step stool with a long attached handle you can hold onto and steady yourself as you climb.
- Wide treads are recommended
- Keep your step stool in a handy place in the kitchen. Too often they end up finding a home in the garage.

• Step stool (Stepladder) with attached handle that
  you can hold while on the step.

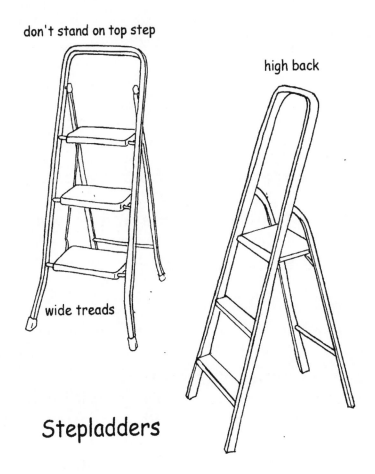

don't stand on top step

high back

wide treads

Stepladders

Handy Gadgets

- **Long handle reacher,** (26-32 inches long)
  Lightweight reachers enable you to grasp items overhead or on the floor without having to bend or stretch. Once you start using this, you will wonder how you got along without it. Available by catalog and some drug stores; see section on catalogs.

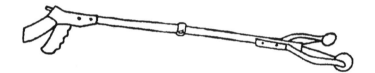

- **Long handle dust pan and broom** eliminates bending.

- **Electric broom or sweeper** makes cleaning easy.

- **Pull out shelving.** Cabinets can be converted to shelving that can be pulled out for easy access.

- **Functional Step Stool** (with long handle) Available from stores such as Target on line and catalogs such as Grandinroad and Sears, see appendix.

- **Kitchen Trolley** a convenient way to transport items. Available in catalogs such as Sammons see appendix.

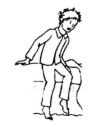

Bedroom

Can your feet touch the floor?

Can Your Feet Touch the Floor?

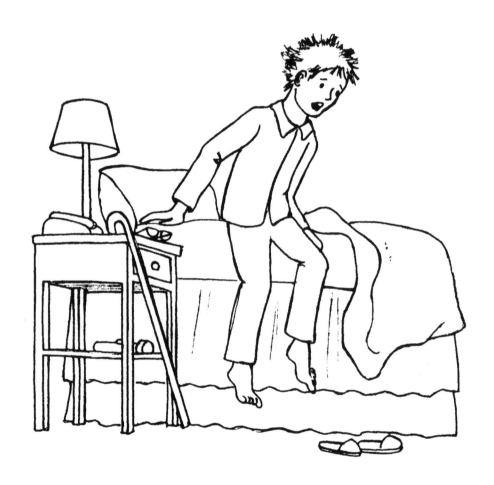

Bedroom

Do you???

- have bedcover/linens that are not slippery
- have a sturdy bedside table with lamp, telephone, flashlight
- have a convenient furniture arrangement
- have clutter free path to bathroom
- have night-lights
- have organized closets
- have a light in your closet
- have an overall bed height that lets your feet touch the floor when sitting on the edge of the bed
- have a mattress in good condition

Hot Spot
Bedroom

The hot spots:
- slippery linens/bedcover
- inadequate lighting
- cluttered bedroom arrangement
- unsafe furniture
- cluttered closets
- old mattress
- bed height too high
- not knowing what to look for when replacing mattress

After twelve years we finally bought a new pillow top mattress. We couldn't wait for it to be delivered! Imagine my surprise when I sat down on it, and my feet couldn't touch the floor! To make matters worse, my old fitted sheets didn't fit. Sound familiar?

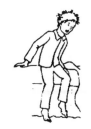

Solution for A Safe Comfortable Bedroom

1. Choose linens that are not slippery. Stay away from slippery satin sheets and glossy comforters.

2. Light a clear uncluttered pathway to the bathroom using cool burning night-lights.

3. Place a sturdy night table next to the bed (avoid three legged tables) with tabletop space for glasses, telephone, tissues, and flashlight. If you use a cane, there is a table cane clip available to hold your cane. Check your local drug store or catalogs. (See handy gadgets.)

4. Use a sturdy chair for dressing.

5. Unclutter and rearrange the shelves and rods in your closet so your most used items are within your range of reach. Lower closet rods as needed. There are many companies who will design and build a closet to your needs or provide do it yourself kits. See appendix.

6. Install a light in your closet; battery powered closet lights are available.

Solution for Bed Height

Your feet should rest flat on the floor when sitting on the edge of the bed. Here are some helpful measurements:

- an overall measurement of about 22 inches from the floor to the top of the mattress should accomplish this if you are of average height
- modern mattresses now measure 8-12 inches deep, a "pillow top" mattress measures 15-18 inches deep
- a box spring is 8 inches deep: a low profile box spring is only 4 inches deep
- a standard bed frame with casters is 8 inches high (keep casters locked to prevent bed from moving) remove casters if bed is too high or consider shortening legs on bed

When buying a new mattress/box spring remember that your height will help determine what you buy to make sure that your feet rest flat on the floor when sitting on the edge of the bed. Usually a 10 inch deep mattress with a four inch box spring on an eight inch high bed frame will do this.

Get a new mattress when:

- your body leaves an imprint in the mattress
- mattress surface begins to look uneven
- mattress creaks when you roll over
- it is 8-10 years old
- read mattress shopping 101

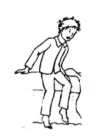

Solution
Mattress Shopping 101

Mattress dimensions:
- Twin   39in. x 75in.
- Twin extra long   39in. x 80in.
- Full   54in. x 75in.
- Queen   60in. x 80in.
- King   76in. x 80in
- California King   72in. x 84in.

The widest bed is two twin beds pushed together. Some people prefer the flexibility of twin beds since they can be pushed together or kept separate, and they are the easiest to make.

According to the Better Sleep Council a box spring and mattress are designed to work together, so purchase them as a pair. A box spring is as important as a good mattress. Don't put a new mattress on an old box spring. For more information see appendix; www.bettersleep.org
Successful comparison shopping is difficult. Go to a reliable company and ask your friends for recommendations.

Solution
Mattress Shopping

At the Store

Before going to the store, measure the height of your existing bed frame and bring the tape measure with you to the store. Remember, an overall measurement from the top of the mattress to the floor should be about twenty two inches: If you are of average height this should enable your feet to touch the floor when sitting on the edge of the bed. This height is the most secure for getting in and out of bed.

When you go to the store wear comfortable clothes and lie down on the mattress (in your usual sleeping position). Don't be in a rush and don't be embarrassed. The experts recommend lying on the mattress for 10-15 minutes in the store. The mattress should gently support your body and evenly distribute your weight. The firmest mattress is not always the best. It is what feels right to you.

When testing out your mattress look at the box spring and frame. Make sure that the total height of your new mattress, box spring and bed frame will allow your feet to touch the floor when sitting on the edge of the bed. To avoid mistakes have the height of the purchased box spring written on the order form and check this on delivery.

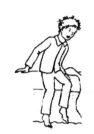

Solution
Hassle free Mattress Delivery

The usual arrangement is the store will deliver and set up your new mattress and take away your used mattress and box spring. If you are not satisfied with your new set it can usually be returned. At the time of purchase have this requirement written on the sales slip.

Now that your new mattress is in place, and you breathe a sigh of relief do not be surprised if the mattress takes <u>a little</u> getting used to during the first week. It should feel wonderful in a matter of days thanks to all the homework you did before buying it.

Handy Gadgets

- **lamp "touch" adapters:** converts any lamp into a touch lamp, touching the lamp will turn it on and off (available in catalogs such as Bruce)

- **cane holder:** allows cane to lean securely on edge of table/desk keeping cane handy and preventing it from falling out of reach (inexpensive gadget found in drug stores and catalogs such as Active Forever see appendix)

- **night-lights:** use cool burning night-lights in bedroom, hallways and bathrooms (night-lights can be a fire hazard if they come in contact with flammable materials, it is best to use cool burning bulbs and keep clear of any fabrics)

- **stand up eye glass case:** lets you find your eyeglasses easily for a safe walk to the bathroom, (available in catalogs such as Gold Violin, Lillian Vernon)

- **closet organizing products and/or a company:** to help you manage your space, and keep your belongings in your range of reach (see appendix)

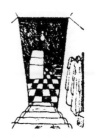

Basement

Dangers Below

Dangers Below

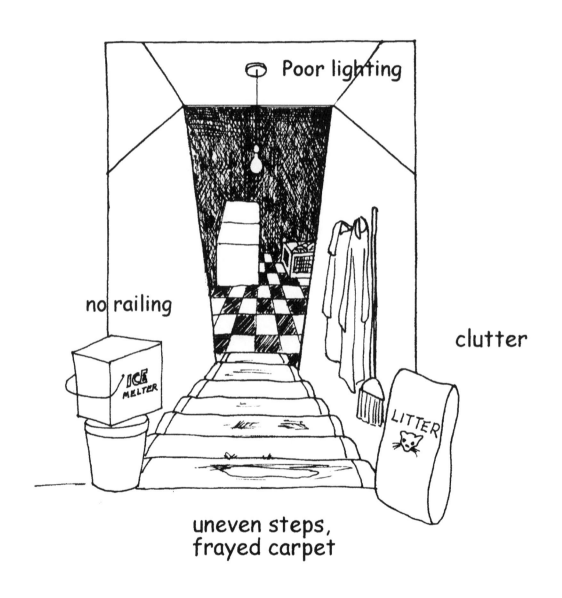

BASEMENT

Are There/Is there???
- a bolt/latch on basement door
- secure stairs
- highlighted stairs
- open tread stairs
- no throw rugs/frayed carpet
- functional secure hand railings
- clutter-free steps
- a well lit stairway and basement
- a light switch at the top and bottom of the stairs
- an available flashlight
- access to a phone
- laundry facilities
- clear path to circuit breaker
- clear path to hot water heater and furnace
- no clutter

Hot Spot
Basement

Hot spots are:
- no bolt/latch on the basement door
- a steep, narrow staircase
- wobbly or uneven steps of varying height
- open tread steps
- insecure and inadequate railings
- using steps to store items
- throw rugs/frayed carpet
- poor lighting
- poor location of appliances
- no accessible phone
- clutter

Maggie was rushing to finish her morning chores. She was meeting her friend for lunch. Before she left the house she wanted to vacuum, wash the breakfast dishes and put the wash in the dryer. After she finished vacuuming, she ran down the basement stairs to put the laundry in the dryer. Slowly she became aware of her husband's distant voice, "Maggie, are you alright?" Maggie opened her eyes and tried to put the pieces together but her arm hurt and why was she lying on the basement floor? Little by little the pieces were put together but not before a trip to the hospital. The diagnosis was a mild concussion, broken wrist and elbow.

Maggie was not holding onto the railing and missed the top step causing her to fall down the basement stairs.

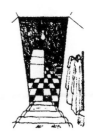

Solution for Basement Stairs

1. Give your basement stairs the same care and attention as your main household stairs.

- Doors that lead to the basement should be latched closed. Guests may assume they are going outdoors and instead end up falling down the basement stairs.
- Highlight the steps with contrasting colored tape. Plastic decorative/repair tape works well. Basement steps often have unexpected unequal heights which cause trips. See Maxi Aids catalog for tape.
- If stairs are open backed have them closed in for safety. If tread is too narrow to close in then highlight each step with white tape or paint.
- Don't place throw rugs at the top or bottom of the stairs; they are a common cause of slips.
- No frayed carpeting.
- Have secure rounded hand railings, preferably on both sides, running the full length of the stairs.
- Don't store items on the steps.

Solution for Basement

Basement stairways can be more hazardous than stairs in the main house; many times they are steep, narrow, poorly lit and have inadequate railings.

2. Brighten up the stairway and basement.
- Have a light switch at the top and bottom of stairs.
- Provide glare-free lighting. Sconces are a good option.
- Use the highest wattage bulb that the fixture allows. We always like to use the full spectrum white lights or fluorescent tubes as these provide bright light.
- Have a flashlight at the entrance to the basement. Install a flashlight holder on the wall.

3. Keep a clear pathway to the hot water heater, furnace, circuit breaker and water shut-off valve.

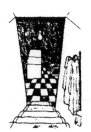

Solution for Basement

4. Washer and dryer
- If your washer and dryer are located in the basement you may want to move them upstairs.
- Today many models of washing machines and dryers are compact and can fit in a closet. This would eliminate carrying laundry up and down the stairs.
- If you must carry laundry on stairs, instead of a laundry basket use a large mesh/canvas tote bag that keeps one hand free to hold onto the railing.

5. Access to phone
- If you use your basement you need to have an accessible phone that can be reached from the floor.

6. Clutter
- Clean out that basement.
- If you don't want anyone to see your basement then you know you have a problem.

Handy Gadgets

- **Washer/dryer** To avoid carrying laundry up and down stairs move washer/dryer to a more convenient location on main living level. If space is a problem consider purchasing a compact washer/dyer unit.

- **Flashlight holder for top of staircase wall** (available at your local hardware store)

- **A Water alarm** is an inexpensive battery alarm that sits on the floor/wall and will beep when it comes in contact with any water. It is useful to place a water alarm near the hot water tank in case of a leak. (available at hardware store and catalogs such as Brookstone's Hard to Find Tools))

- **Tote bag for carrying laundry** Until you relocate your washer/dryer you can use a tote bag to carry laundry which will free a hand to hold the railing and will not obstruct your vision.

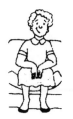

Furniture

Does it fit?

Does It Fit?

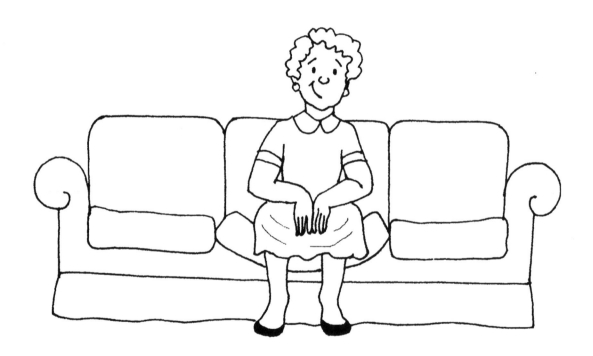

Furniture

Chairs/Sofas

Do you/Can you???
- have chairs without casters/wheels
- rest your feet on the floor when seated
- know what to look for in a chair/sofa
- sit with ease
- stand up easily
- have helpful furniture-armrests that extend the full length of the chair

Tables/Furniture Location

Do you have???
- a coffee table that is not a tripping hazard
- a glare free coffee table top
- a sturdy table next to your chair
- a rocking chair positioned with runners out of the walking path
- a three to four foot uncluttered pathway through main traffic areas

Hot Spot
Poor Fit of Furniture

We all have experienced the middle cushion of an overstuffed couch and the embarrassment of not being able to stand up or sit down gracefully.

Hot spots are:
- no armrests
- armrests that don't extend the full depth of the seat
- soft, sinkable cushions
- seat depth too deep
- seat height too low
- lack of firm back support
- wide recliners
- recliners that are difficult to operate
- chairs with wheels/casters
- coffee tables that are too low
- glass top tables that cause glare
- three legged tables-they tip over easily
- too much furniture
- a rocking chair

When the fit of your furniture encourages a slouched posture with your head and shoulders slumped forward, that can become the posture you will have when you stand. Poor posture is a contributing factor to falls.

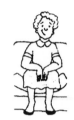

Solution for Furniture

1. What to look for in a chair and sofa...
- armrests that extend at least the full depth of the seat
- a stable base in chairs and sofa
- no wheels
- seat cushions that offer good support
- firm back support
- proper seat height, not too low (if it is too low, it is more difficult to stand up)
- proper seat depth (if it is too deep, it is more difficult to stand up)

The best test to determine the proper fit of furniture is to sit in the chair with your buttocks all the way back in the seat. Your feet should be flat on the floor and have about one inch clearance from the chair to the back of your knees. This should be comfortable, and you will be able to stand up with ease.

See illustration on next page.

Illustration of a sturdy chair: Notice how the armrests extend the full length of the seat.

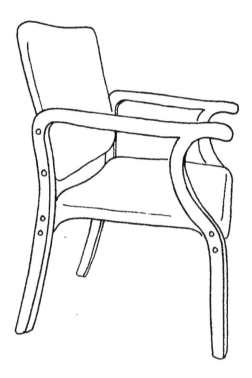

Width of the seat...... at least 18 inches
Depth of the seat......16 to 20 inches
Height of chair seat ..15 to 17 inches from the floor
Height of arm rest......7 ½ inches from the chair seat

Solution for Furniture

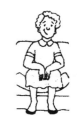

2. What to look for in recliners...
- recliners are not one size fits all
- women usually require a narrow recliner
- narrow recliners make it easier to reach the hand control
- some have a seat lift mechanism (see handy gadgets)

3. What to look for in a coffee/end tables...
- low coffee tables are a tripping hazard
- glass inserts cause problems with glare and depth perception, use a cloth runner on glass table top to prevent this problem
- do not use three legged tables, light weight tripod tables tip over easily

4. What to look for in furniture placement: We have a mental picture of our home in our minds and rearranging the furniture can cause unexpected trips.
- store small footstool under the coffee table to prevent tripping over it when you are not using it
- place rocking chair runners out of the path of traffic to prevent tripping over them
- remove all unnecessary furniture and clutter, you want a three to four foot uncluttered pathway

Handy Gadgets

- **Lumbar support roll or back hugger pillow**-reduces seat depth and provides support.

- **Support under seat cushion to take away sag**-makes it easier to stand and encourages good posture when sitting. (Available through catalogs such as Lillian Vernon and Home Trends, see appendix)
- **Furniture risers**-go under furniture legs to make sofa higher.(Available in catalogs and stores such as Bed, Bath and Beyond)
- **Couch cane**-a hand railing that is anchored by the weight of the couch. A couch cane can act as an assist when standing up from a low couch. (Available in catalogs such as YouCan TooCan, see appendix)
- **Portable seat lift mechanism**- seat that assists you to stand and can be moved to any chair. Recliners can be purchased that have the mechanism installed. (Available at surgical supply stores and catalogs such as Active Forever, see appendix.)
- **Armrest Pockets**- Cloth pockets that drape over the arm rests that hold the remote control, TV guide, tissues and other necessities.(Available in catalogs such as Gold Violin and Lillian Vernon)

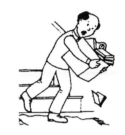

Stars

Do you know where you're headed?

Do You Know Where You're Headed?

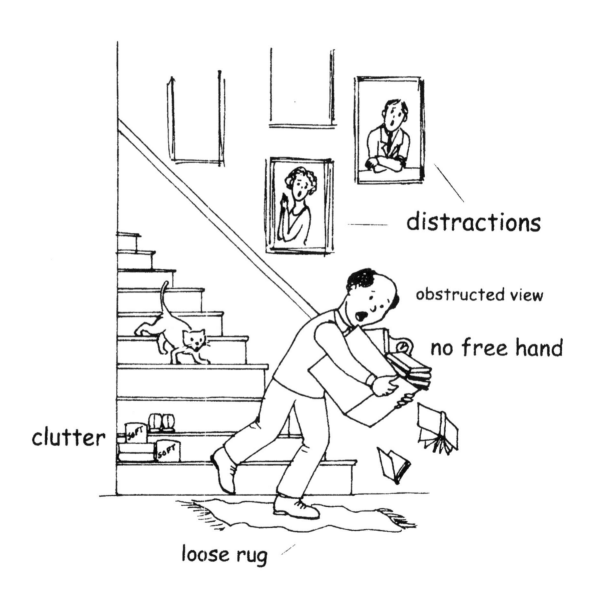

Stairs

Are there/Is there???

- sufficient tread width
- uniform riser height
- railings on both sides
- railings that extend beyond the entire length of stairs
- highlighted stairs
- low pile carpeting on the stairs
- no throw rugs
- non-slip bare stairs
- no open tread stairs
- a light switch at the top and bottom of the stairs
- no articles placed on stairs
- no distractions on stair walls

Hot Spot
Stairs

Hot spots are:
- narrow treads
- unequal riser heights
- no railing/insecure railing
- plush carpeting/loose carpeting
- dark color carpeting
- throw rugs at landings
- bare stairs
- open treads
- spiral staircases
- one and two step stairs
- no highlighting on stairs
- inadequate lighting/glare
- clutter and distractions
- distortions in depth perception
- attic stairs

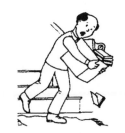

Solution for Stairs

1. Always do a **"Quick Mental Step Check"** before you go up or down stairs that you are not familiar with. Check for...

   - railings -do they run the full length?
   - height   -are they all the same height?
   - nosing   -is there an overhang?
   - surface -do they look slippery?
   - carpet   -is it thick, frayed or loose?
   - lighting -can you see the stairs clearly?
   - glare   -does it affect your vision?

2. **Techniques to use when you encounter unsafe stairs:**
   - use the hand railings
   - take one step at a time
   - go up the stairs with your strong leg leading
   - go down the stairs with your weak leg leading (the strong leg is actually holding you as you go down the stair)
   - if there is only one banister place both hands on the railing and go up/down sideways

Ideal Stairs

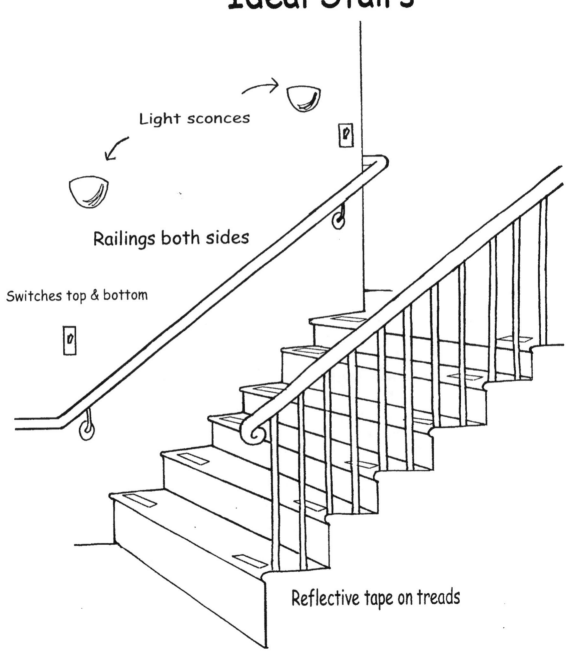

Light sconces

Railings both sides

Switches top & bottom

Reflective tape on treads

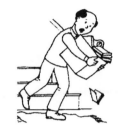

Solution for Stairs

3. Functional Hand Railings need to be
- secure and on both sides of the stairs
- extend beyond the full length of the stairs
- rounded with adequate wall clearance to provide a good hand grip

4. Shallow Tread (depth of stair): Take special care to place your <u>whole foot</u> on the tread of the stair.
- stair tread should be at least 11 inches deep
- 11 inches allows the foot enough room to rest safely on the step without hanging off
- treads less than 9 inches can result in a missed step
- to put this in perspective a woman's size 7 shoe is 9 inches long

5. Highlight Stair Treads
- highlight steps with reflective or contrasting color tape
- a ¼ inch variation in riser height can cause a misstep (riser is the height of the step)
- variation in height of riser is most often seen in one and two step stairs-highlight with contrasting tape

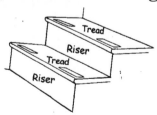

Solution for Stairs

6. Carpeting

- All carpets tend to blur the edges of the stairs making it difficult to see where one step ends and the other begins. This is especially true with dark colors. Highlighting the edge of each step with contrasting color tape will solve that problem.
- Avoid patterned carpets because they can interfere with depth perception and cause a misstep.
- Stair runners need to be fastened securely and not worn or frayed.
- Thick carpeting on stairs can cause a trip because it interferes with sensory feedback from our feet. (This sensory information helps our balance.)
- Plant each foot carefully when you encounter plush carpeting. We recommend a low dense tight-weave carpet.

7. Throw Rugs

- Never place throw rugs by stairs—they can skid out from under you.
- We like to say throw out your throw rugs! If you insist on keeping them, make sure they are securely attached to the floor with double-sided tape and/or anti-slip material. (Available at hardware stores.)
- Throw rugs that are placed on top of carpet can creep, bunch up and cause a trip. See section on floors.

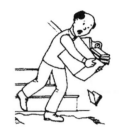

8. Bare Stairs

For decorative purposes many people prefer to keep their stairs bare. Bare stairs can be slippery, produce glare, and their edges can blur together causing falls.

We have found the following solutions to be effective:
- Paint the stair tread and riser different colors.
- Paint just the edge of each step.
- Use white or colored tape at the edge of each step.
- Use a matte finish to reduce glare and slippery surface.
- ALWAYS hold onto railings. Make this a habit!

Gail's mother had the creative idea to use different colored carpet treads on her bare stairs. This proved to be a pretty way to distinguish each step. If you do this make sure they are securely fastened. She used carpet tacks and the mats have stayed in place for 20 years!

9. Open Tread Stairs
- Special care is needed when using open tread stairs because without the backboard it becomes difficult to judge depth and foot placement.
- If there is sufficient depth (tread) we recommend getting a carpenter to close these. Until then highlight step edges, use railings and step carefully!

10. Spiral Stair Cases
- Use both railings!
- If possible convert them to something safer.
- At a bare minimum close in the backs.

11. One and two step stairs

Often we have heard, "I only have one step into my family room." Our experience has shown that it is that step that causes a fall.

- Falls occur on one or two step stairs because; they are usually unexpected, have varying heights, may have an overhang and don't have railings.

- All safety factors that apply to a full flight of stairs are even more important with one or two step stairs.

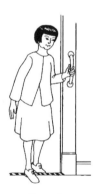

- All one and two step stairs need adequate lighting, railings and highlighting.

- If there isn't enough room for a railing then at least install a safety hand grip. Safety hand grips are available in catalogs such as Bruce, see appendix. See picture.

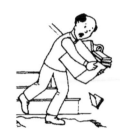

Solution for Stairs

12. Lighting/Vision

- Make sure steps are well lit the entire way.
- Have light switches at both the top and bottom of the stairs.
- Check and correct for any glare. Glare interferes with vision and can cause misjudgments in steps. Wall lighting (sconces) helps reduce glare. See main section on lighting.
- Use maximum recommended wattage.
- Changing light bulbs and cleaning light fixtures can be a special problem on stairs; get someone to do this for you.
- Take special care on stairs when wearing eyeglasses; especially if you are a new wearer of progressive/multi-focal glasses. Be aware that where you look through the lens can change depth perception and cause misjudgment in the height and depth of the stair. Bifocals can also cause distortions when going down stairs. If you encounter this problem don't just accept it; talk to your optometrist.

Solution for Stairs

13. Clutter/Distraction

- Don't use stairs as a storage center. It's a common practice to place items on the steps. This is a bad habit that has caused many falls as we trip on them because we forget they are there.
- Don't allow the cat or dog to sleep on or by the stairs.
- Be aware that pictures hung on walls along staircases can distract you and cause a fall. Look at the step and not at the pictures when you are climbing and descending stairs.

14. Attic Stairs

- Don't use pull down attic stairs.
- Avoid the attic if it has not been made into a living area with proper stairs and telephone.
- Have family members help take inventory and relocate seasonal items from attic to an accessible area.

FYI: A stair glide can be installed in your home if you can no longer negotiate stairs safely. This option can be rented or purchased and providers of this equipment can be found in the yellow pages under the heading 'mobility companies'.
As people look to their future some new homes are being built with elevators.

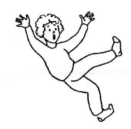

Floors

Whoops!

Whoops!

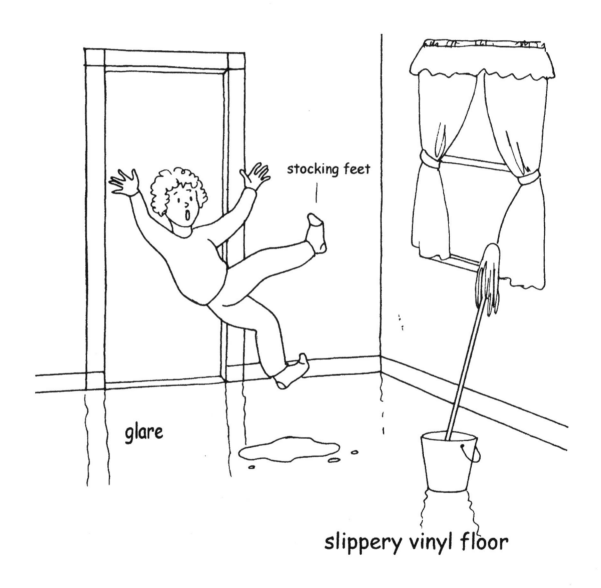

stocking feet

glare

slippery vinyl floor

Floors

Are there/Is there???

- secured throw/scatter rugs
- secured area or oriental rugs
- thick wall to wall carpeting
- buckle-free carpeting
- no frayed or worn carpets
- non-slip coating on tiled or marble floors
- slip-resistant linoleum/vinyl
- matte finish on hard wood floors
- glare free flooring
- even thresholds
- no electrical cords stretched across the floor
- no clutter

Hot Spot
Floors

Hot spots are:
- throw rugs
- area rugs
- thick carpeting
- wet tiled floor
- newly waxed linoleum floor
- high gloss slippery finish
- thresholds greater than ½ inch
- electric cords
- clutter

Barbara was washing the kitchen floor. As she backed out of the kitchen she remembered she left her newspaper on the counter. She took off her shoes thinking her stocking feet wouldn't dirty the drying floor and went back to get her newspaper. She slipped on the wet floor and broke her hip.

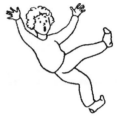

Solutions for Hazardous Floors

A uniform floor surface eliminates thresholds and is easiest to walk on.

1. Throw Rugs

- People are charmed by throw rugs and don't realize they pose a serious threat. Throw rugs cause trips and slips and we recommend removing them completely.
- Throw rugs placed on top of a carpet buckle and move. That bunched up rug will knock you off your feet!

2. Area Rugs

- Large area rugs need to have rubber backing or non-slip backing placed underneath them.
- The ends of the rug can be secured to the floor with double-sided tape.
- Fringe, tassels and shag styles can cause trips.

Solutions for Floors

3. Carpeting
- Thick carpeting is difficult to walk on.
  Have you noticed that your feet don't feel as "grounded" on plush carpet? This is because plush carpet reduces the sensory feedback needed for balance.
- When it is time to replace the carpet, shop for carpeting that is made of a low, tight pile. This is easier to walk on and care for.
- Avoid densely patterned carpets; they can distort depth perception. We recommend a solid color carpet which contrasts with the wall color.
- Carpets can stretch with age and this leads to buckling. Replace the carpet or have it re-stretched to eliminate this tripping hazard.

4. Thresholds (including bathroom)
- To avoid tripping use beveled thresholds.
- Thresholds higher than ½ inch need to be removed or tapered.

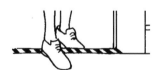

- All thresholds should be highlighted with tape.

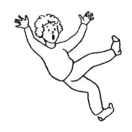

Solution for Floors

5. Tile Floors

- A tile floor is very slippery when wet and a hard unforgiving surface to land on.
- Since most bathroom floors are tiled, we recommend a low pile wall-to-wall bathroom carpet that has rubber backing and is mold resistant. The carpet will absorb any dripping water; provide firmer footing and a warm soft surface.
- If you are unable to replace a slippery tile floor then have it treated with a non-slip coating. (available at your local hardware store)

6. Vinyl or Linoleum Floors

- If you are redoing a bathroom or kitchen floor stay away from ceramic tile or stone floors. They are hard, cold and slippery.
- Consider a vinyl or linoleum floor. They are softer and easy to clean. Check its coefficient of friction, or COF. A COF measures how slippery a floor surface is. A COF of 0.6 or higher is generally considered a slip-resistant floor.

Solutions for Floors

7. Wood Floors (use proper non-slip cleaning products)
- Wood floors are easy to walk on provided they don't have a high gloss slippery finish. A matte finish prevents glare and slipping. Never clean floors with furniture polish; it will turn your floor into a slippery bowling alley floor.
- When area rugs are used on top of wood floors make sure there is rubber matting underneath the whole rug, or secure the rug to the floor with two-sided tape.

8. Electric Cords on the floor
- Keep your cords neat and out of the way. Make sure electrical cords are not placed so they are a tripping hazard.
- Never place electric or extension cords under carpeting.
- If you find that you are using extension cords have your electrician put in additional outlets. The most convenient height for an outlet is 27 inches from the floor.

9. Clutter
- Keep a three to four foot uncluttered pathway through main traffic areas.
- Keep old newspapers and magazines to a minimum and off the floor!
- Magazines and newspapers are very slippery when stepped on.
- When cleaning keep canister vacuums out of pathway.

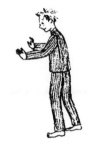

Lighting

Bumps in the Night

Bumps in the Night

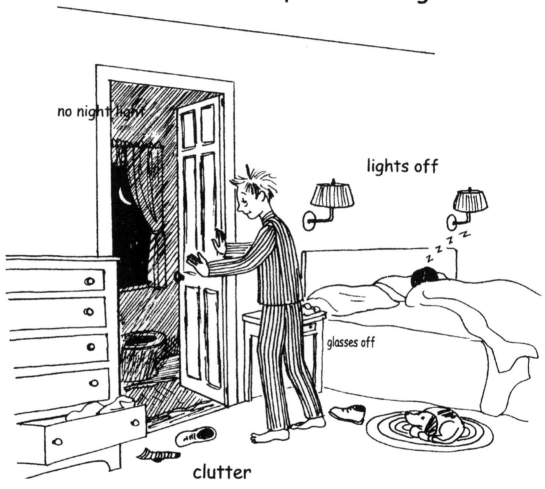

no night light

lights off

glasses off

clutter

LIGHTING

Are there/Is there???
- good lighting throughout house
- a light switch at the room's entrance
- light bulbs with maximum allowed wattage
- smooth transition lighting from room to room
- cool burning night-lights in all bathrooms, bedrooms, hallways
- electrical timers controlling lights
- a light switch at the top and bottom of the stairs
- glare free lighting
- translucent window shades/sheer curtains to reduce glare
- sufficient electrical outlets

Hot Spot
Poor Lighting

To read, adults older than 50 require 3 to 5 times more light than a younger person.

It also takes a longer for adult eyes to adjust to different levels of light. For example, coming into the house from the bright outdoor sunshine can cause "temporary blindness". Give your eyes time to adjust.

Hot spots are:
- not enough lighting
- lighting that produces glare
- entering a dark room

Keep those lights on! The money you are saving is minimal at best and is not worth a fall. You have to see it to avoid it.

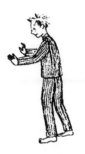

Solution for Poor Lighting

1. Provide adequate lighting

With aging it is considered normal for eyes to need more time to adjust to different levels of light. We have all experienced that temporary feeling of blindness when walking from the sunny outdoors into a darker room.

- check the light fixtures to make sure they are clean
- check to see that light bulbs have the maximum wattage allowed
- keep a lamp on a timer so you won't enter a dark room
- have a light switch at the top AND bottom of stairs
- have your electrician install more outlets, light switches and/or lighting if needed

    A convenient height for electrical outlets is 27 inches from the floor but others prefer 18 to 30 inches. Decide what is best for you.
- place cool burning night-lights in all bathrooms, bedrooms and hallways

Solution for Lighting

2. Glare

Glare is a villain because it interferes with vision and can cause temporary blindness.

Ways to reduce glare:

- Translucent fabric shades will let light in the room while reducing glare.

- Sheer curtains help reduce glare.

- Opaque lampshades should cover any bare bulbs.

- Indirect lighting from wall sconces on stairway walls will reduce glare.

- Light colored walls brighten a room without producing glare.

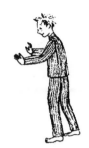

Solution

3. Entering a dark room

- Have light switch at room entrance.

- Make sure that light bulbs can be changed easily.
  Some fixtures are designed so that the casing
  doesn't have to be removed. Other fixtures may be
  covered by a large dome/globe that can be difficult
  to handle.

- Replace flip switches with illuminated rocker
  switches, these are easier to see and to turn on.
  Until you replace switches use reflective tape on
  existing switches so they can be seen in the dark.

- Place lamps on a timer so you never have to enter a
  dark room.

- Take both night-lights and a flashlight with you
  when you travel.

Handy Gadgets

Night-lights are available in many different sizes, colors and styles and can be easily found in food stores, hardware stores, department stores, etc. Use cool burning bulbs to reduce the chance of fire if bulb comes in contact with curtains, pillows or bedspreads. Take night-lights with you when you travel, they help light up an unfamiliar room.

Illuminated light switches eliminate the need to feel your way along the wall to the light switch. Simply change the switch plate from a flip to an illuminated rocker switch. No special wiring is necessary. (Available at hardware stores)

Auto-touch lamps
Any lamp can be converted into an auto-touch lamp by plugging the lamp into a simple conversion device. Then all you have to do is touch any metal part of the lamp to turn it on and off. (Available in catalogs such as Bruce.)

Power emergency lights
These small lights are a little larger than the average night-light and stay plugged in all the time but they only light up when the power goes out. (Available at hardware stores and catalogs such as Lillian Vernon.)

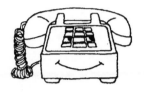

Telephone

Where I Need to Be

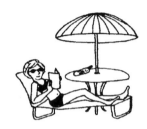
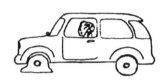

Where I Need to Be

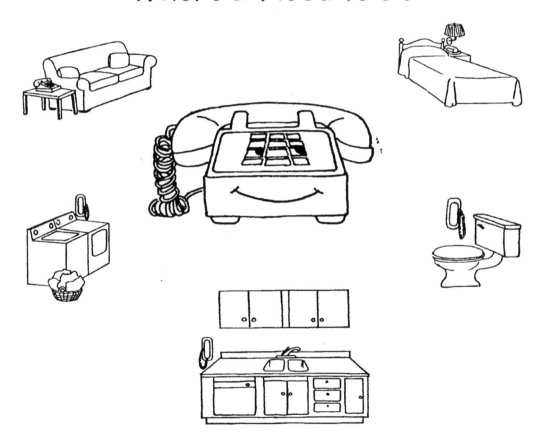

telephone

Are there/Is there???

- several accessible phones
- a cordless phone
- phones that meet your needs
- memory buttons
- an answering machine
- a cell phone

Hot Spot
No Accessible Phone

Many falls occur when rushing to answer a ringing telephone.

Hot spots are:
- not enough telephones in the house
- no accessible phones
- no answering machines
- a long dangling telephone cord

Elizabeth was vacationing at a lovely resort hotel. Following her tennis game she returned to her room to shower before lunch. She slipped on the wet bathroom floor and could not get up. Fortunately a reachable phone was right there and she got immediate help for her sprained ankle. After this experience Elizabeth decided to have one installed in her own home bathroom.

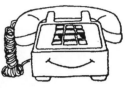

Solution for No Accessible Phone

1. **Place phones in the most frequently used rooms**: kitchen, bedroom, TV room and bathroom.

2. **Phones should be placed so they can be reached from the floor**. We have heard many stories from our patients about being unable to reach a phone after a fall.

3. **Install a phone in the bathroom and basement or get in the habit of bringing one in with you**.

4. **Have a least one standard phone.** In a power failure a cordless phone doesn't work.

5. **Have a cordless phone** that you carry with you to the basement and out in the yard.

6. **Cordless phones** replace the need for long dangling cords that are a tripping hazard.

7. **Cell phones** need to be regularly charged and if you have one practice using it or you might forget how to use it.

8. **Multi-pack phones** include a base phone and convenient add-on phones that don't require a jack.. See handy gadgets.

Handy Gadgets

- Amplification device to increase volume for those with poor hearing. Give your phone company a call to learn what services they provide for decreased hearing and low vision.
- A large number pad makes it easier to dial.
- An electronic voice announces each number to ensure correct dialing.
- Programmable one-touch memory buttons for emergency and frequently dialed numbers.
- Answering machine eliminates the need to rush to a ringing phone.
- Caller ID allows you to know who is calling before answering the phone.
- Multi-pack phones (corded or cordless) that require only one phone jack for the main phone and come with other phones that only need an electrical outlet to work.
- TracFone, prepaid cell phone that does not require a monthly plan. Available at most discount department stores.

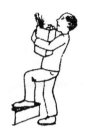

Garage

No Wonder I Trip

No Wonder I Trip

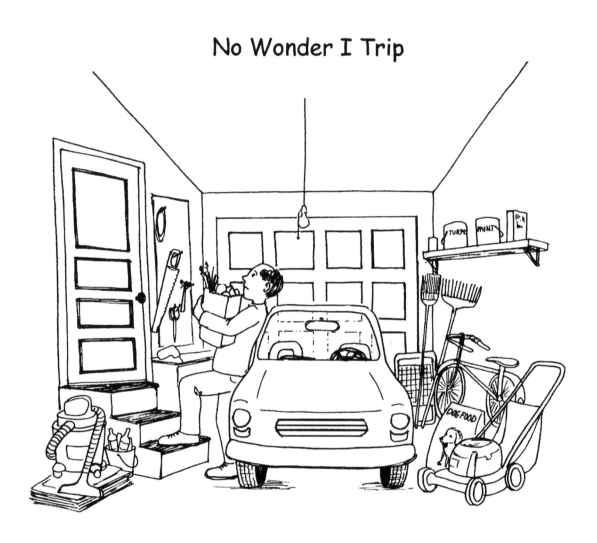

Garage

Are there/Is there???

- adequate lighting
- a garage door opener
- a clean clutter-free garage
- no oil spills/drippings
- sturdy stairs
- highlighted steps
- secure stair railings

Hot Spot
Garage
**Garages are full of fall hazards. Garages tend to become
a catchall for odds and ends. In addition they usually
have poor lighting, cluttered pathways, slick spots and
unfinished stairs without a railing**.

Hot spots are:
- inadequate lighting
- heavy sticky garage doors
- accumulated treasures/clutter
- oil drippings
- poorly constructed steps
- no hand railings
- wobbly hand railings

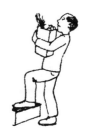

Solution
Garage

1. Let there be light!
- use maximum allowed wattage in all light fixtures
- keep all light fixtures clean
- have light switches at all entrances into the garage
- have a flashlight by the garage entrance
- if the garage is detached, use motion detector lighting to light up the pathway to the house

2. Garage door openers:
- are a necessary convenience that eliminate the lifting of heavy doors and provide short term lighting when operated
- offer easy access into homes with an attached garage
- do not work during a power failure, so understand how the pull down release works so that the door can be operated by hand
- make sure the safety rebound feature functions and reverses the motion when it touches an object under it
- have a garage door company inspect them yearly

Solution
Garage

3. Clutter control
- have a garage sale to clear out unused items
- establish a clear pathway through your garage
- wipe up oil spills/drippings
- there are clutter control companies who will organize your garage

4. Watch those steps!
Garage steps are often neglected. All stair safety measures need to be applied to garage steps as well!
- hand railing on each side
- even risers-any uneven risers need highlighting tape on the treads
- well lit
- step edges marked with contrasting tape

Treat all steps with care!

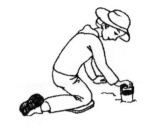

Deck/Garden

Outdoor Living

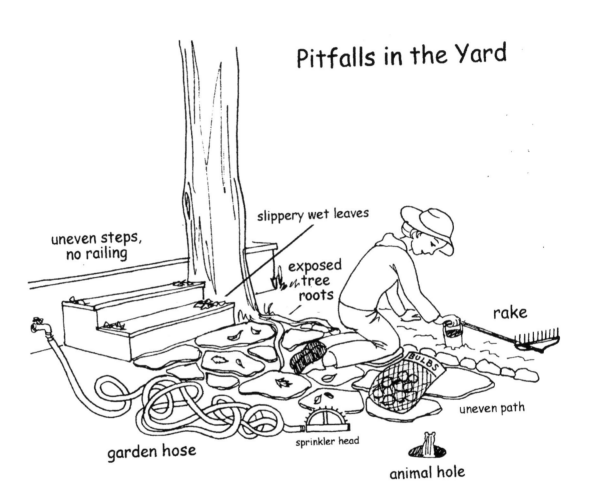

Pitfalls in the Yard

uneven steps, no railing

slippery wet leaves

exposed tree roots

rake

garden hose

sprinkler head

uneven path

animal hole

94

Outdoor Living

Garden

Do you have/use???
- no hidden tripping hazards
- light weight easy to handle equipment
- proper body mechanics when bending and lifting
- regular tree maintenance to remove fallen branches and dead wood

Patio/Deck

Do you have???
- a wooden deck
- a flagstone patio
- a cement patio
- a brick paver patio

Hot Spot

Nature fills our gardens and yards with tripping hazards.

Hot spots are:
- uneven surfaces
- tree roots
- critter holes
- slippery surfaces
- sun glare
- no telephone
- cumbersome equipment
- equipment not put away
- poor planning
- poor body mechanics
- deck/patio stairs

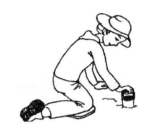

**Solution
Outdoor Living**

1. Check Your Walking Surface

- Make sure outside paths, patios and decks are level and smooth. Eliminate uneven surfaces. See section on walkways.
- Until uneven surfaces are repaired, highlight the raised surface with a small strip of white paint.
- Use white spray paint to highlight critter holes, tree roots and protruding sprinkler heads that are in your path.
- Be wary of wet leaves, wet grass, slushy snow, ice and the dreadful black ice on all surfaces including decks. Have ice melt on hand or stay home. Do not attempt to walk on ice. Keep ice melt handy in a closed container by your front door, back door and garage.
- Algae growth on wooden decks can be very slippery. Power washing usually rids the deck of algae.
- Remember to use sunglasses to cut down on glare. Be careful when re-entering the house/garage, remove sunglasses and give your eyes time to adapt to the new level of light.

Solution
Outdoor Living

2. Replace cumbersome/outdated equipment. Check out your garden supply store for new designs in garden tools. We like the following:
  - light weight coiled hoses
  - light weight flower pots
  - padded long handle garden tools
  - light weight wheel barrows
  - padded kneeling surface with arm rails

Available in catalogs such as Active Forever, see appendix.

3. Put all equipment away in its proper place.
  - Put tools and hoses away when you are done with them. We have all been guilty of leaving our hose/rakes draped across the pathway.

4. Plan Ahead For Low Maintenance Gardening.
  - Plan for the convenience of raised beds and container gardening.
  - Consider a hiring a lawn service (and snow plowing for winter). Walking on uneven lawn surfaces is challenging enough without pushing a lawn mower.
  - Keep trees trimmed to prevent fallen branches.
  - Gail's British mother-in-law made a plan to gradually change her garden to a lighter maintenance perennial garden, including slow growing shrubs. She also used raised beds that enabled her to garden in comfort without bending.

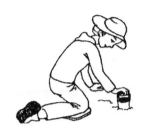

Solution
Outdoor Living

5. Body Mechanics To Keep You On Your Feet

- Good posture and lifting rules need to be followed when carrying heavy pots and soil.
- Don't carry a load so large that it obstructs your vision.
- Use a wagon to help transport plants.
- Heavy items need to be held close to your body.
- Lift with your legs not with your back. This means that you bend down by bending your knees not by leaning over.
- Use padded kneeling bench with arm supports which help you stand up. Available at garden stores.
- Remember there are lightweight pots available today.

6. Take Your Cell/Cordless Phone With You...

- Then you're not tempted to hurry inside to answer the phone.
- Then you won't miss that important call.
- Then you can always make a call.

Solution
Outdoor Living

7. Highlight Stairs

- Multi-tier decks are beautiful but shadows can cause missteps. We recommend highlighting all steps.
- Highlight all deck stairs that have unequal risers.

While visiting his parents, Gail's 24 year old son had the unfortunate experience of missing the last step on their new deck stairs and sprained his ankle. The last stair blended in with the landing. This step edge is now highlighted with white paint and highlighting tape.

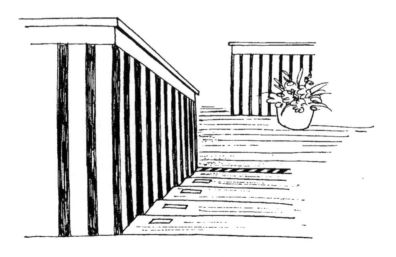

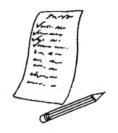

Home Repairs

Check it Out

Check It Out

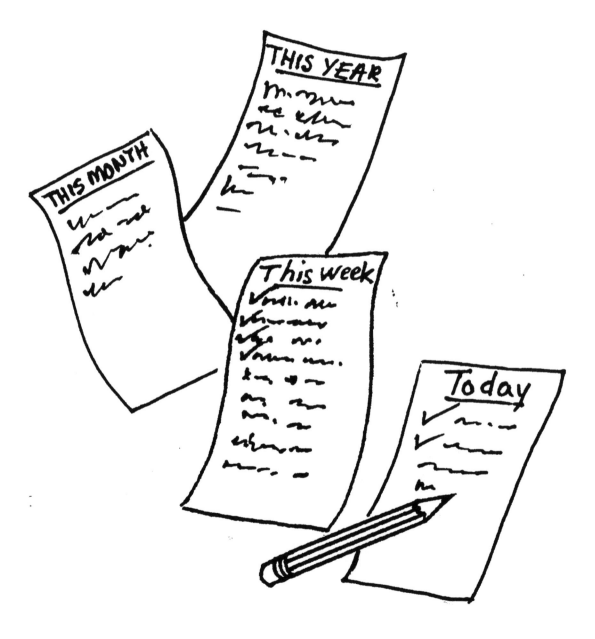

Home Repairs

Do you ???

- make household adaptations and repairs to allow you to age safely at home
- keep a list of repairs for: Today
  This Week
  This Month
  This Year
- know where/how to hire a contractor, handyman, or other licensed professional
- think that you cannot afford home repairs
- know what universal design is

Hot Spot
Procrastinating on Home Safety Repairs

Hot Spots:
- putting off safety repairs
- not having a repair plan
- not having a trusted repairman
- not having a financial plan for home repairs
- being penny wise and pound foolish

FYI The cost of one to two months in a nursing home/assisted living facility equals the cost of updating your bathroom.

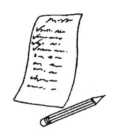

Solution
Home Repairs

Don't let your house kick you out!
Make a To Do List Today!

- Use the safety checklist located on page 119 to help identify your personal home safety hot spots.
- Start with a shopping list of things you need to buy. Example; light bulbs, highlighting tape, answering machine, phone.
- Prepare your work list of things to do; today, this week, this month, this year.

Solution
Finding a Repairman

Steps for finding trustworthy repairmen.
- ask friends, neighbors, workers at local hardware stores and senior centers for recommendations
- check to see that the repairman is licensed if plumbing or electrical work is required
- check with your better business bureau for any complaints
- ask for and check with local references
- ask for written estimate
- ask if the repairman is insured
- never give approval to go ahead with a job until you have thought about it for a day or two

Walk away from repairmen if:
- they request full payment before work begins
- they can not provide local references for recent work
- there is nothing in writing
- there is no business address
- plumbers/electricians can't produce a license

Often the best work is done by local repairmen. They depend on their reputation and can be easily contacted after the work is completed.

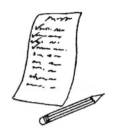

Solution
For Major Renovations

- Think user friendly and universal design when planning any major renovation.

- Universal designs are solutions that can be useful for all ages. For example, a lever door handle can be opened easier than a round one both by arthritic hands and small children's hands. Consider using universal design when planning new construction.

- AARP is one resource for information on universal design. You can also find Certified Aging in Place Specialists (CAPS) who are trained in modifications that help people continue living safely and independently at home. For information on finding CAPS see AARP or National Association of Home Builders (NAHB) in appendix.

Solution
For Financial Concerns

- Call your local Department on Aging and ask what services, loans or reduced rates for home modifications are available for older persons.

- Call your local senior citizen center and ask them what programs there are that help older persons with home repairs and chores.

- You do not know what help is available until you spend some time researching it.

- Request repairs as a birthday/holiday gift. See appendix for list of suggestions.

- For major renovations talk to your bank about home equity loans or reverse mortgages. AARP has information on financing home repairs.

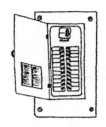

Home Emergencies

Be Prepared

Be Prepared

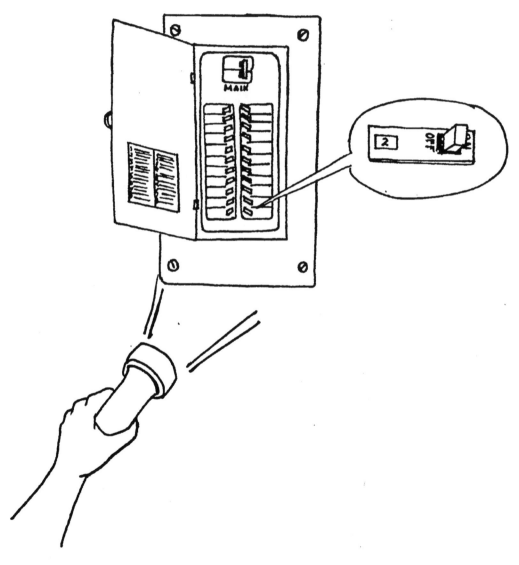

Home Emergencies

Do you ???
- know how to turn off main water supply
- know where your circuit breaker is
- have emergency phone numbers next to phone
- have a fire escape plan
- have a small portable fire extinguisher and understand how to use it
- have a smoke detector and carbon monoxide detector on every floor
- have a water/flood alarm
- have flashlights with batteries
- have spare batteries
- have a power failure safety light
- have a battery operated radio
- have one standard/corded phone

Hot Spot
Being Unprepared

Hot spots are:
- not having proper supplies
- not knowing location of supplies
- panic and confusion during an emergency
- not having read directions for any emergency equipment including fire extinguishers and carbon monoxide detectors

Solution
For Home Emergencies

Be Prepared!

1. **Everyone in the house needs to be prepared for emergencies.** Being prepared will prevent panic and rushing that can lead to a fall.

   - **Know where the main water valve** is and how to turn it off. It's usually located where your water meter is. If you don't know where it is, call your water company.

   - **Place water/flood alarm** near hot water heater, it will alert you when there is a leak. This is an inexpensive bell shaped alarm that attaches to the wall and will ring when it detects water. (Available at Brookstone Hard to Find Tools Catalog see appendix)

   - **Know where your circuit breaker is.** Usually they are located in the basement or the garage. Make sure there is a clear path and a flashlight nearby.

   - **Have smoke alarms and carbon monoxide detectors** on each floor, replace batteries twice a year.

   - **Have a fire escape plan** that is practiced by all family members. Include a location to meet outside the home.

   - **Keep a list of all your important phone numbers next to the phone and programmed into cell phone.** Remember 911 is your emergency number.

Solution
For Home Emergencies

2. Have emergency supplies gathered together in a handy place.
- Have a fire extinguisher on each floor. Place one in the kitchen. Read information on how to use them.
- Have flashlights with extra batteries. This eliminates the need to use candles.
- Have power lights that are always plugged into electrical outlets and they will automatically provide light during a power outage.
- Have a battery-operated radio.

3. Have at least one standard corded phone. Cordless phones don't work during a power outage. If you have a cell phone make sure it is kept fully charged.

The main idea is to prevent panic and rushing that could lead to a fall.

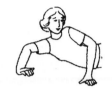

What To Do If You Fall

Take Inventory

What to do if you fall.

1. Take a deep breath and take inventory, make sure you are not injured. If you are not injured, roll onto your side. (If you are injured use your fall pendant or reachable phone and call for assistance.)

2. Get onto hands and knees.

3. Crawl to a sturdy chair or couch; a low piece of furniture will provide the best support. If chair seat is too high you can always place hands under the cushions.

4. Use both your arms and legs to push up and then stand.

5. Turn around and sit on the chair or couch.

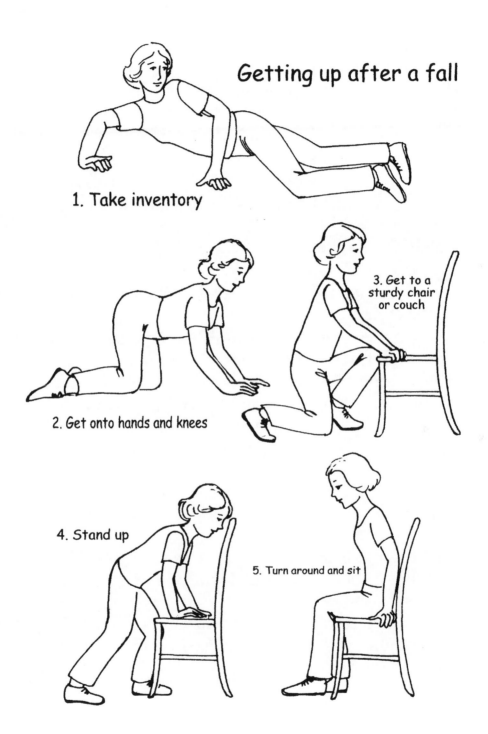

Getting up after a fall

1. Take inventory

2. Get onto hands and knees

3. Get to a sturdy chair or couch

4. Stand up

5. Turn around and sit

117

What to do if you are unable to get up:
- there is no rush
- take a deep breath
- determine what hurts
- use your accessible phone
- if you are using a fall pendant then push the button and help will come

Fall Pendants:
- provide security
- can be worn as wrist watch, necklace, or clips on the belt
- when activated it notifies a response center who then contacts a pre-designated doctor, family member or friend
- some companies that supply pendants include:
  American Medical Alarms 1 800 542-0438
  Medical Alert Alarm System 1 800 906 0872
  Life Alert 1800 815-5922

Also contact the Red Cross or local Senior Citizen Center as they can provide information and cost on availability.

FYI Some towns have a daily check in call for those who live alone. Check with your local police department.

You have now identified and eliminated fall hot spots throughout your home. Here is a review of the major points for home safety.

Home Safety Review
70 Point Checklist

Entrance: Do you have.....
1. clear and level pathways?
2. secure and highlighted outdoor steps?
3. secure hand railings on both sides of the steps?
4. easily managed door knobs, locks, and storm doors?
6. adequate lighting and motion detector lighting ?
7. an easily accessible mailbox?

Bathroom: Do you have.....
8. grab bars by the toilet and bath/shower area?
9. anti-slip tape or anti-slip surface on shower/bath floor?
10. a secure toilet seat at a comfortable height?
11. night-lights with a cool burning bulb?
12. an available phone?

Kitchen: Do you have....
13. storage within your range of reach?
14. a non-slip floor and a non-slip mat by the sink?
15. step stool with functional handle and wide tread?

Bedroom: Do you have.....
16. a bed that allows feet to touch the floor when sitting?
17. non-slip linens?
18. cool burning night-lights?
19. a clear path to the bathroom?
20. a flashlight on bedside table with extra fresh batteries?

Home Safety Review

Basement: Do you have...

21. a latched basement door?
22. well lit uncluttered stairs in good repair?
23. highlighted stairs with secure railings on both sides?
24. your washer and dryer in the most convenient location?
25. an accessible phone?

Furniture: Do you have...

26. sturdy tables? (no three legged tables)
27. coffee tables that are not too low to be a tripping hazard?
28. glass tabletops covered with a runner to reduce glare?
29. furniture that fits your body?

Stairs: Do you have...

30. highlighted unequal riser heights?
31. highlighted one and two step stairs?
32. highlighted steps?
33. well lit stairs?
34. a light switch at the top and bottom of stairway?
35. uncluttered stairs, no stored items on steps?

Home Safety Review

Floors: Do you have....

36. beveled thresholds or highlighted thresholds?
37. slip resistant floors?
38. secured scatter rugs?
39. carpets in good repair, not frayed or buckled?
40. glare free floors?
41. electrical cords out of walkways and not under rugs?

Lighting: Do you have....

42. light switches at all room entrances?
43. even-lighting in all rooms?
44. use bulbs with the highest recommended wattage?
45. night-lights in all bathrooms, bedrooms and hallways?
46. night-lights that use a cool burning bulb?
47. a flashlight on all levels of your home?
48. a power failure safety light?

Telephone: Do you have...

49. an accessible phone in every room?
50. at least one cordless phone?
51. at least one landline/corded phone?
52. an answering machine?
53. a list of emergency numbers by your phone and programmed into cell phone?

Home Safety Review

Garage: Do you have...
54. stairs in good repair, highlighted with railings?
55. bright lighting?
56. uncluttered floors?
57. automatic garage doors with emergency reverse?

Deck/Garden: Do you have.....
58. good body mechanics when you garden?
59. deck stairs highlighted?
60. secure railings by your deck stairs?

Home Emergencies: Do you know...
61. how to turn off the main water supply?
62. where your circuit breaker is?
63. a fire escape plan?
64. if your smoke alarm/carbon monoxide detector works?
65. where to place a water alarm?
66. if your battery operated radio and flashlight work?
67. to place emergency phone numbers next to phone?
68. an accessible fire extinguisher and know how to use it?

Home repairs: Do you have...
69. a contractor who is familiar with universal design?
70. a plan and timeline for home repairs?

**Start today. Make your home repair notebook:
Projects for today, this week, this month and this year.**

Congratulations. This is a good start to your fall prevention program but it is only half of the solution. To be effective in preventing falls you need to also address your body and life. We recommend you read the companion book; *Fall Prevention: Stay On Your Own Two Feet!*

Fall Prevention: Stay On Your Own Two Feet! provides solutions for physical and lifestyle changes that may contribute to falls.

Topics include:
- Balance
- Posture
- Strength
- Exercise
- Fear of Falling
- Vision
- Medications
- MD Relationship
- Shoes/Feet
- Clothing
- Pets

****

To order additional copies of this book or the companion book,

Fall Prevention: Stay On Your Own Two Feet! ISBN 0-7414-3239-0
go to www.buybooksontheweb.com and enter fall prevention
or go to **www.amazon.com**

Or call Toll-free 877 BUY BOOK (877 289-2665)

Visit our website: www.fallpreventionadvisors.com

To Do List

1

2

3

4

5

6

7

8

9

10

11

12

13

14

Appendix

When your family and friends ask you what you would like for your birthday, never say, "I have everything I need." Instead take a look at the following lists for some ideas.

List of Gifts

Answering machine
Bath bench/shower chair
Big button telephone programmed with emergency numbers
Carbon monoxide detector
Cell phone
Central vacuum system
Chair that fits your body
Coiled light weight garden hose
Cool burning night-lights
Comfort height toilet
Companion Volume, *Stay On Your Own Two Feet!*
Electric broom
Electrical timers for lights
Elevated toilet seat
Flashlight with extra batteries
Floor gripper for area rugs
Garden kneeling bench
Grab bars
Hand held shower
Large key turner, provides extra leverage for easy turning
Lever door handles
Lightweight fire extinguisher
Lightweight flower pots
Lightweight vacuum cleaner
Long handle dustpan
Long handle reacher
Long handle shoehorn
Mattress (proper height)
Motion sensor lighting
Pill organizer

Portable phone
Reflective, white and plastic coated colored tape
Rolling garbage cans
Step stool with tall hand railing
Sturdy bench by front door for packages
Timer for lights
Trolley cart/kitchen cart
Visit to a physical therapy clinic for establishing an exercise/balance program
Washer/dryer compact appliance
Water alarm
Water temperature/anti-scald valve
Window treatments that reduce glare
YMCA/YWCA membership

List of Services/Repairs

Additional light switches where needed
Change batteries in smoke alarms and carbon monoxide alarms twice a year
Change flip switches to rocker switches
Clean out basement, garage and attic
Highlighting of stair edges with tape
Install anti-scald device
Install lever door handles
Install lever faucets
Install garage door opener
Install secure hand railings on all stairs
Install shower head with slider bar
Lawn care
Personal fall alarm system
Professional installation of grab bars
Relocating laundry room from basement to main level
Repairing cracked driveways/walkways
Replace raised thresholds with beveled thresholds
Secure existing hand railings
Snow removal
Upgrade light fixtures for easy access
Window washing

Additional Books

Accessible Gardening: Tips & Techniques for Seniors & the Disabled, Joann Woy, 1997.

Aging in Stride, Christine Himes, M.D., Elizabeth N. Oettinger, M.Div. Dennis E. Kenny, J.D. 2004.

The Complete Guide to Alzheimer's Proofing your Home, Mark L. Warner, 2000.

Elderdesign: Designing and Furnishing a Home for Your Later Years, Rosemary Bakker, 1997.

Elder House: Planning your Best Home Ever, Adelaid Altman, 2003.

Home Planning for Your Later Years, William K Wasch,, 1996.

Home Sweet Home: How to Help Older Adults Live Independently, Dennis R. La Buda, M.A. and Vicki Schmall, Ph.D, 2000.

How to Avoid Falling: A Guide for Active Aging and Independence, Eric Fredrikson, 2004.

How to Care for your Aging Parents, Virginia Morris, 2004.

How to Prevent Falls: A Comprehensive Guide to Better Balance, Betty Perkins-Carpenter, 1993.

Merck Manuel of Heath and Aging: The Comprehensive Guide to the Changes and Changes, 2005.

Popular Mechanics Home Safety Handbook: Practical Tips for Safe Living, 2005.

Helpful Catalogs

We do not endorse any of the following products or catalogs. We are including them for the reader to investigate and decide what fits their individual needs. Items, phone numbers and web sites do change but to the best of our knowledge were accurate at the time of writing.

Active Forever www.activeforever.com 1 800 377-8033 They include items such as walk-in bathtubs, bath lifts, reachers, cane holders, portable seat lifts, shower benches, and stair glides.

AliMed www.alimed.com 1 800 225-2610 The Help At Home catalog has health care products for the lay person.

Bathroom systems: There are many companies that provide modular shower units and walk in baths. You can speak to your plumber and get materials from such companies as:
> **Best Bath Systems-** www.bestbath.com 1 800 727-9907 A.
> **Independent Living USA** www.independentlivingusa.com 1 800 403-7409
> **Premier Baths** www.primier-baths.com 1 800 578-2899
> **Safety Tubs** www.safetytubs.com 1800 250-7832

Brookstone Hard to Find Tools and Brookstone Tools www.brookstone.com 1 800 926-7000 Includes non slip reversible chair pads, night lights and a water alarm sensor.

Bruce Medical Supply www.brucemedical.com 1 800-225-8446 They carry many helpful products including the small "grab-it" handle and "auto touch lamps".

Closet Organizing Systems There are companies who build and organize closets and kitchens using universal design. For the do-it yourself person there are kits available. Such companies include:
> **California Closets** www.californiaclosets.com 1 888 336-9709
> **EasyClosets.com** www.easyclosets.com 1 800 910-0129

Are You Organized? www.areyouorganized.com 1 203 775-2991 (systems for the home handyman or woman)
Closet Maid www.closetmaid.com 1 800 874-008 (systems for the home handyman or woman)

Diadot Disability Solutions www.diadot.com 973 875-5669 Providers of colored nylon grab bars.

Doctors Foster and Smith www.drsfostersmith.com 1 800 826-7206 Helpful gadgets for your pets to prevent them from being "underfoot".

Fall alert devices. (Personal Emergency Response Systems) We recommend checking with your local Red Cross, senior center, police department, or county office on aging they may have resources for obtaining fall alert devices.
There are many companies that provide fall alert devices including:
    Medical Alarm/ Medical Alert System www.medicalalarm.com 1 800 906-0872
    Lifeline www.lifelinesystems.com 1 800 543-3546
    Lifestation www.lifestation.com 1 800 884-8888

Functional Solutions (North Coast Medical) www.BeAbleToDo.com 1 800 821-9319 Products include dressing aids, exercise equipment, and a selection of bath aids that includes a folding shower bench for travel.

Gold Violin www.goldviolin.com 1 877 648-8400 Products include colorful shower chairs, stylish canes, and walkers etc.

Grandinroad www.grandinroad.com 1800 491-5194 Carries a step stool/ladder with a functional handle and other household items.

Home Trends www.hometrendscatalog.com 1 800 810-2340 Home products including a cushion seat support.

Improvements www.improvementscatolog.com 1 800 642-2112 Provides products to make life easier in the home, garden and car.

Klein Design Inc. www.kleindesign.com 1 800 451-7247 Mail order furniture company.

Lillian Vernon Catalog www.lillianvernon.com 1 800 901-9402 They provide useful household gadgets including a power outage light.

MaxiAids www.maxiaids.com 1 800 522-6294 A good resource for many products including low vision, low hearing, and highlighting tapes.

Products for Seniors www.productsforseniors.com 1 800 566-6561
A website that offers senior friendly products including outdoor non- slip strips to put on slick concrete walkways or steps.

QVC television www.qvc.com 1 800 345-1515 Independent living products can be seen and ordered on their "In Home Care Show" (see QVC's program scheduling)

Sammons Preston www.sammonspreston.com 1 800 323-5547 The Enrichment catalog is geared to the lay person. Carries Wingit Grab Bar Fastening System.

Sears Health and Wellness Catalog, 1800 326-1750 Aides for daily living.

SeniorShops www.seniorshops.com 1 800 894-9549 They have over 900 products targeted to seniors including a detachable cylinder pill organizer.

Target Store www.target.com Carries some senior friendly products including a functional two step stool.

Walter Drake www.drake.com or 1 800 525-9291 Many useful gadgets including extra long tub mats and cushion supports.

YouCan TooCan www.youcantoocan.com 1 888 663-9396. Has many products to make life easier including a couch cane that is used as an assist when standing up from a low couch.

Helpful Organizations

Administration On Aging www.aoa.gov 202 619-0724 Click on Elders and Families and choose any of the topics on services, healthy lifestyle or resources. To reach your local offices call 1 800 677-1116, or call your local town hall or senior center. Your local office provides information on such things as home repair programs, tax rebates, fall pendants, support groups and aging in place programs.

AARP www.aarp.org 1-888 687-2277 This is a useful resource for information about housing, safety, fall prevention and aging successfully. Click on Health, then click Staying Healthy and then click Health Guide to useful links on aging. AARP provides some free publications including, The *Do-Able Renewable Home; Make Your Home Fit Your Needs*, Physical *Activities Booklet* and *Relationships With Your Physician.*

American Diabetes Association: www.diabetes.org 1 800 342-2383 They provide helpful information and education on living with diabetes.

American Occupational Therapy Association (AOTA) www.aota.org 301 652-2682 or 1 800 377-8555. Click on consumer information. The site provides practical information on how to find an occupational therapist in your area who could assess your individual needs and home adaptations. The site also provides links to many specific disease related sites and organizations.

American Physical Therapy Association (APTA) www.apta.org 1 800 999-2782. This organization can help find a physical therapist in your area including physical therapists with specialty certifications in areas such as orthopedics, neurology, and geriatrics.

American Society On Aging www.asaging.org 1 800 537-9728 Offers information on aging.

Arthritis Foundation www.arthritis.org 1 800 568-4045 Offers answers to questions and free brochures about arthritis.

Better Sleep Council www.bettersleepcouncil.com Provides ideas for getting a better nights sleep and information for buying a mattress.

Children of Aging Parents www.caps4caregivers.org 1 800 227-7294 A national nonprofit organization whose mission is to assist caregivers with reliable information on healthcare. The site provides health related links.

Elderweb www.elderweb.com This website contains a database of organizations, and a library of articles, reports, news, and events on senior topics.

Firstgov.gov www.firstgov.gov 1 800 333-4636 Topics for and about senior citizens. Click on the link for citizens for information on aging
.

Home Safety Council www.homesafetycouncil.org 202 330-4900 A site dealing with home safety concerns. Their mission is to educate people of all ages to be safe in and around their homes.

Lighthouse International (vision connection) www.lighthouse.org 1 800 829-0500 212 821-9200 Useful for finding products and information for low vision.

National Association of Professional Geriatric Care Managers www.caremanagers.org 1 520 881-8008. This organization can help locate a geriatric care manager in your area. A geriatric care manger organizes and over-sees needed care giving services.

National Association of Home Builders(NAHB) www.nahb.org 301 249-4000 This organization provides information on universal design when remodeling. They provide names of local builders who are Certified Aging in Place Specialist (CAPS). For a complete list of their publications and cost contact NAHB.

National Council on the Aging www.ncoa.org 202 479-1200 An organization dedicated to improving seniors' lives. This site includes useful links.

National Kitchen and Baths Association www.nkba.org 1 800 843-6522 This organization is a nonprofit trade association which provides resources for consumers and industry professional who need assistance in kitchen and bathroom design or remodeling projects.

National Institutes of Health/National Institute on Aging www.nih.gov/nia 1-800-222-2225. Provides answers to questions on health and aging. They will send you a free booklet, *Exercise: A Guide from the National Institute on Aging.*

National Institutes of Health, Osteoporosis and Related Bone Diseases www.osteo.org 1-800 624-2663 Upon request they will send you a free copy of their brochure on bone health.

National Parkinson Foundation, www.parkinson.org 1 800 327-4545 They will provide free booklets on dealing with parkinson's disease.

National Resource Center, www.homemods.org and also www.stopfalls.org , both sites provide housing information with pertinent links.

****

To order additional copies of this book or the companion book,

Fall Prevention: Stay On Your Own Two Feet!
Go to www.buybooksontheweb.com and enter Fall Prevention

Or call Toll-free 877 BUY BOOK (877 289-2665)

Visit our website: www.fallpreventionadvisors.com

****

Made in the USA
Lexington, KY
17 October 2016